Nurse Jim's Helping Hands

by

J. S. Warner

Illustrations by

Bonnie L. Ferguson

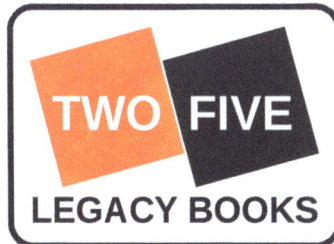

TWO FIVE
LEGACY BOOKS

Published by Two Five Legacy Books,
  An imprint of Warner House Press, USA

Visit: www.jswarnerauthor.com

Disclaimer:
This work is largely a product of fiction. However, School Number 2 is a real place, and the character of Nurse Jim is based on a real person. All other characters and events are fictional, and any resemblance to actual persons, living or dead, is purely coincidental.

Published 2024
Printed in the USA

ISBN: 978-1-951890-57-5

10 9 8 7 6 5 4 3 2 1

For Maria

My Wife

My Love

My Hero

My Everything

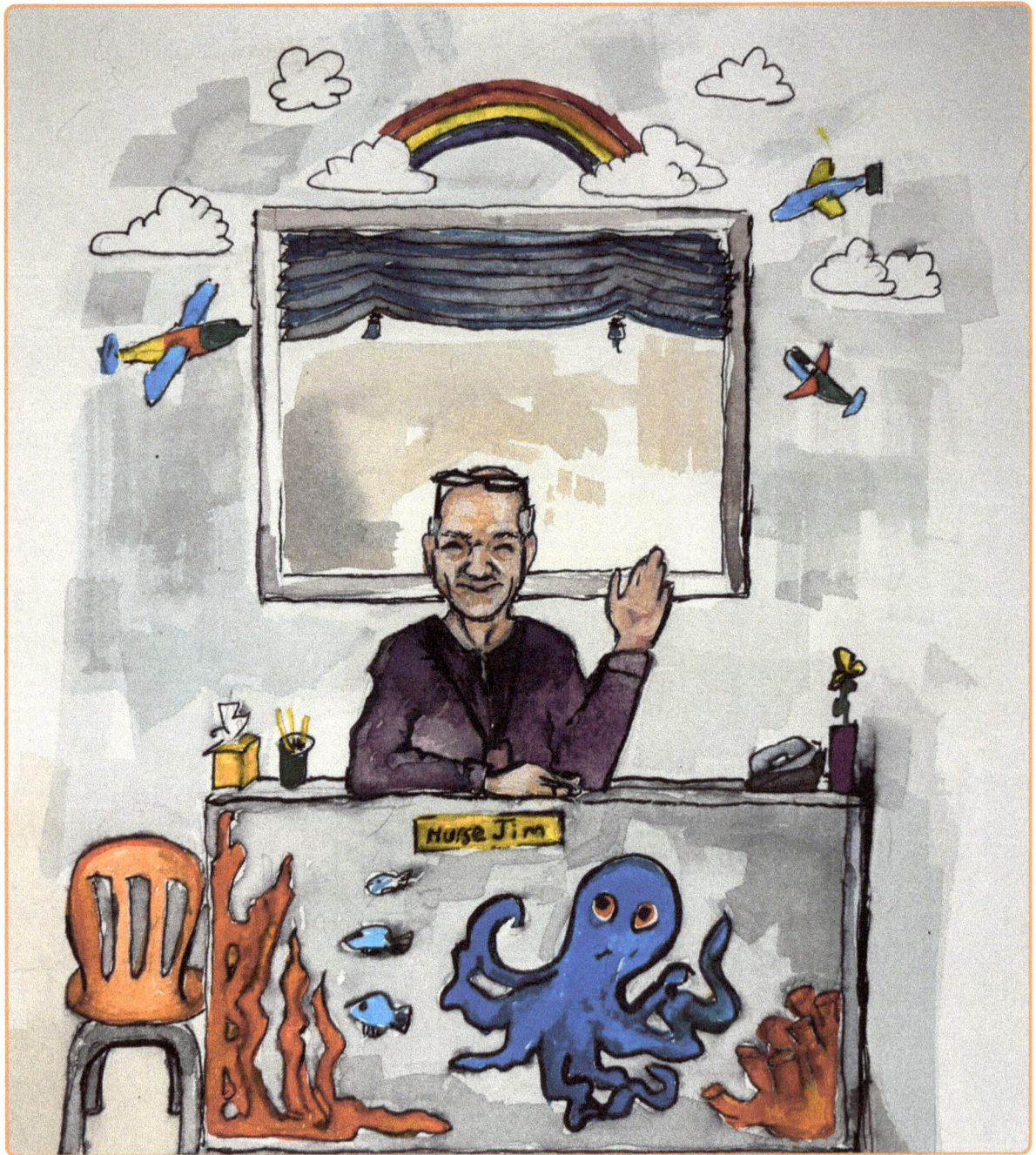

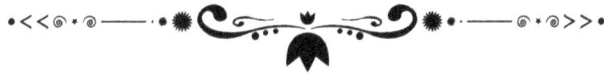

Welcome to School Number Two,
where every child is welcomed by the
friendly face of Nurse Jim in a cozy
office filled with colorful murals.

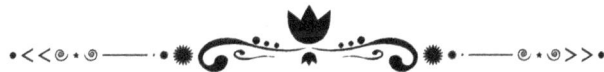

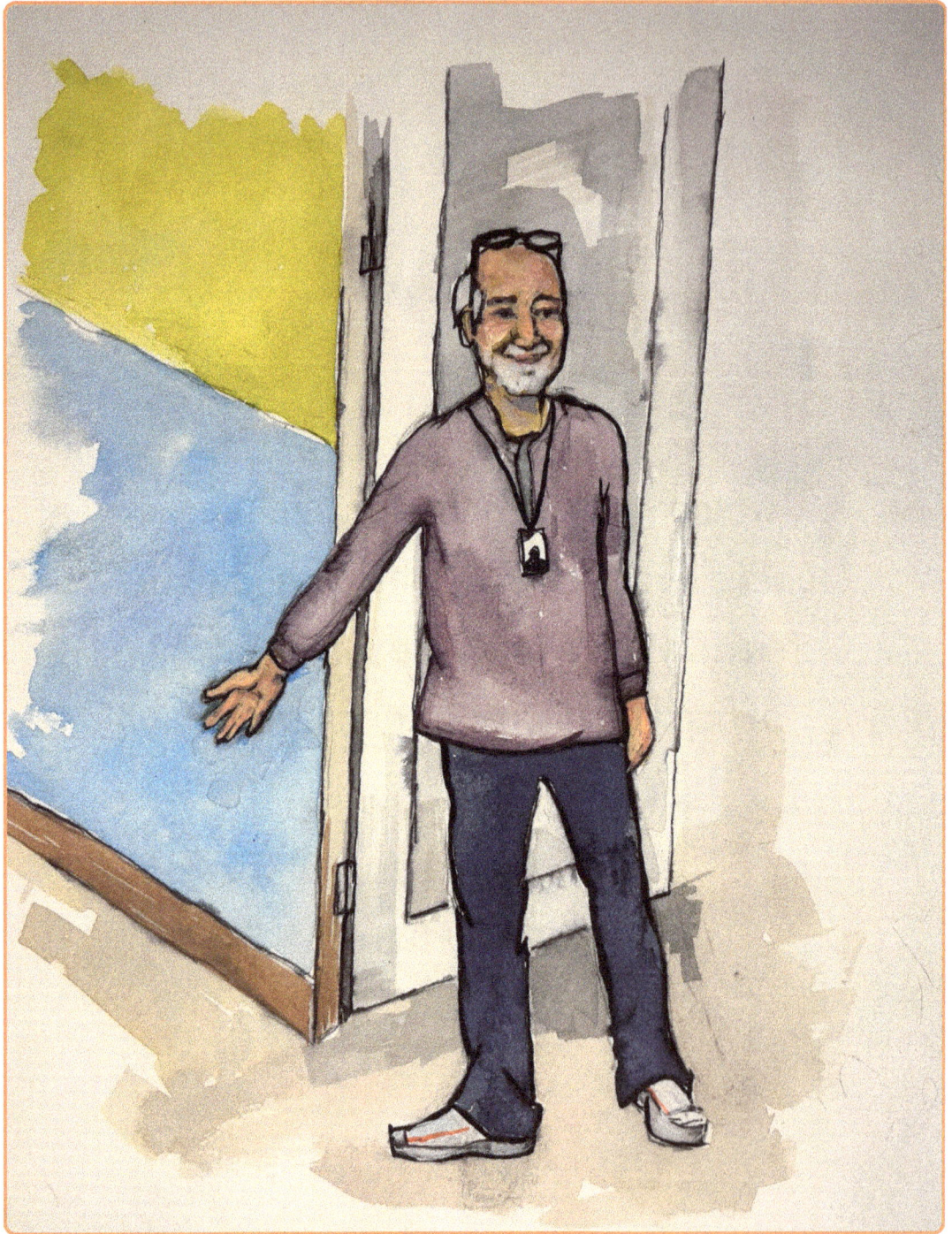

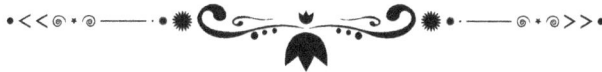

Every morning, Nurse Jim welcomes
the students with a warm smile
and a friendly greeting as they
make their way to class.

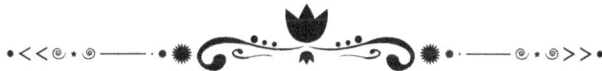

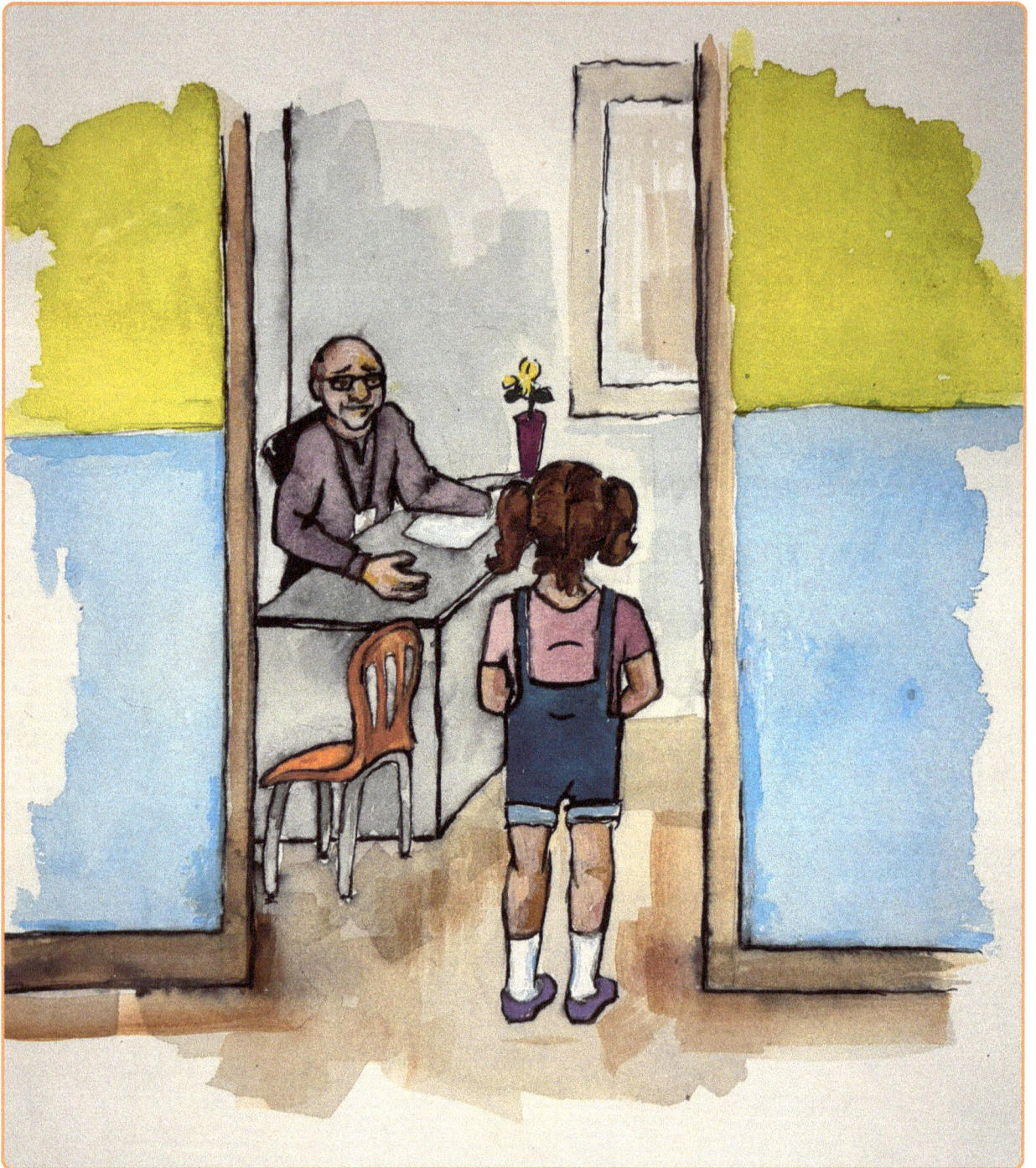

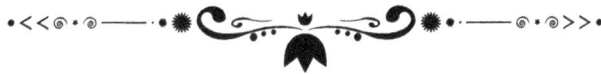

One sunny morning, during recess time,
a young girl named Natalie hurried into
Nurse Jim's office with tears in her eyes.

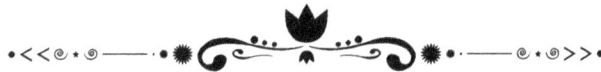

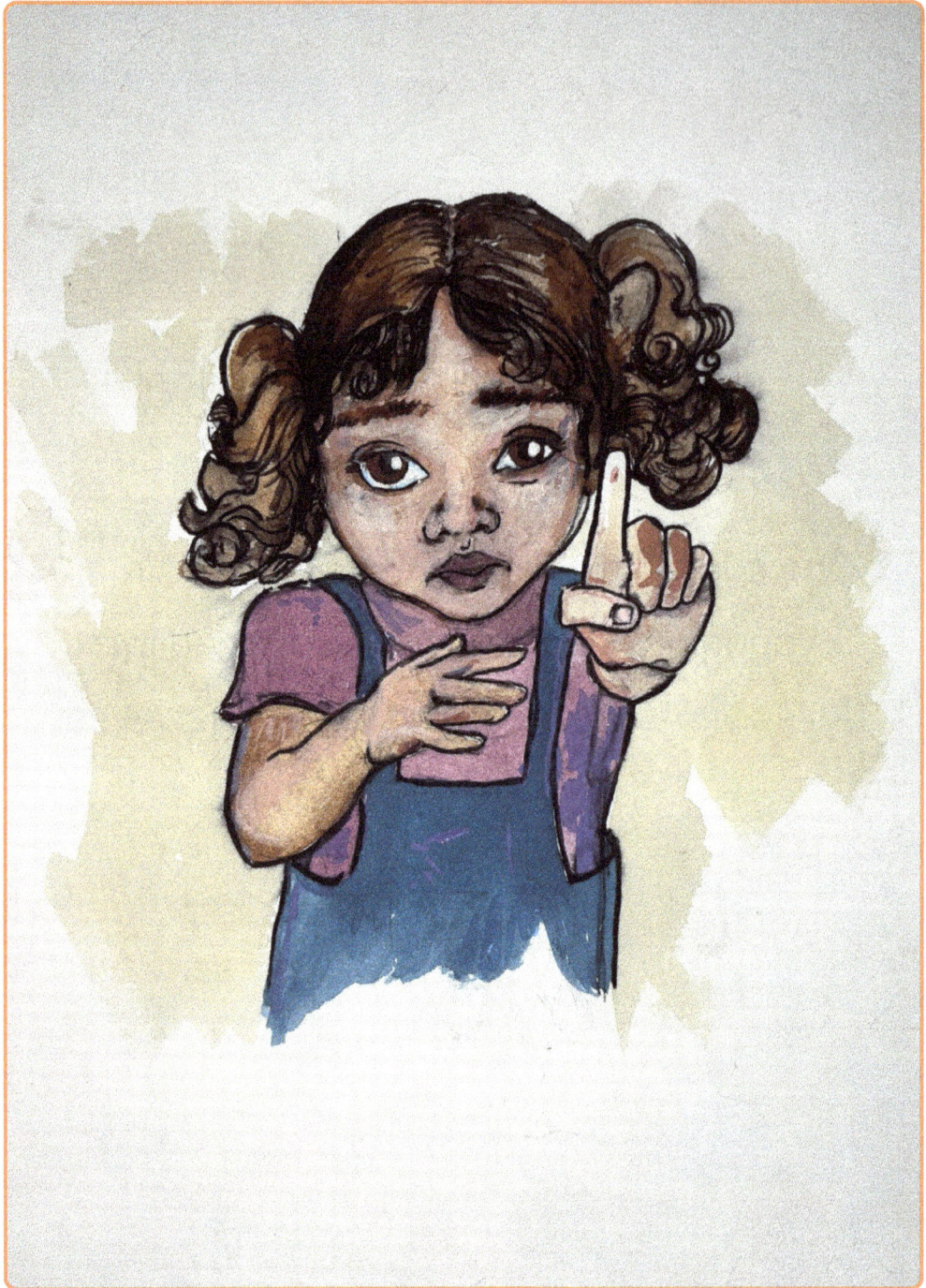

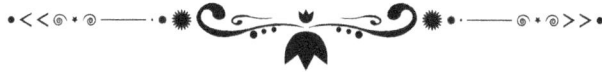

"What's wrong, Natalie?"
Nurse Jim asked.

Natalie sniffled as she extended her
hand, revealing a small splinter.
"I got this from the playground,"
she said with a whimper.

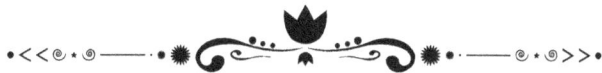

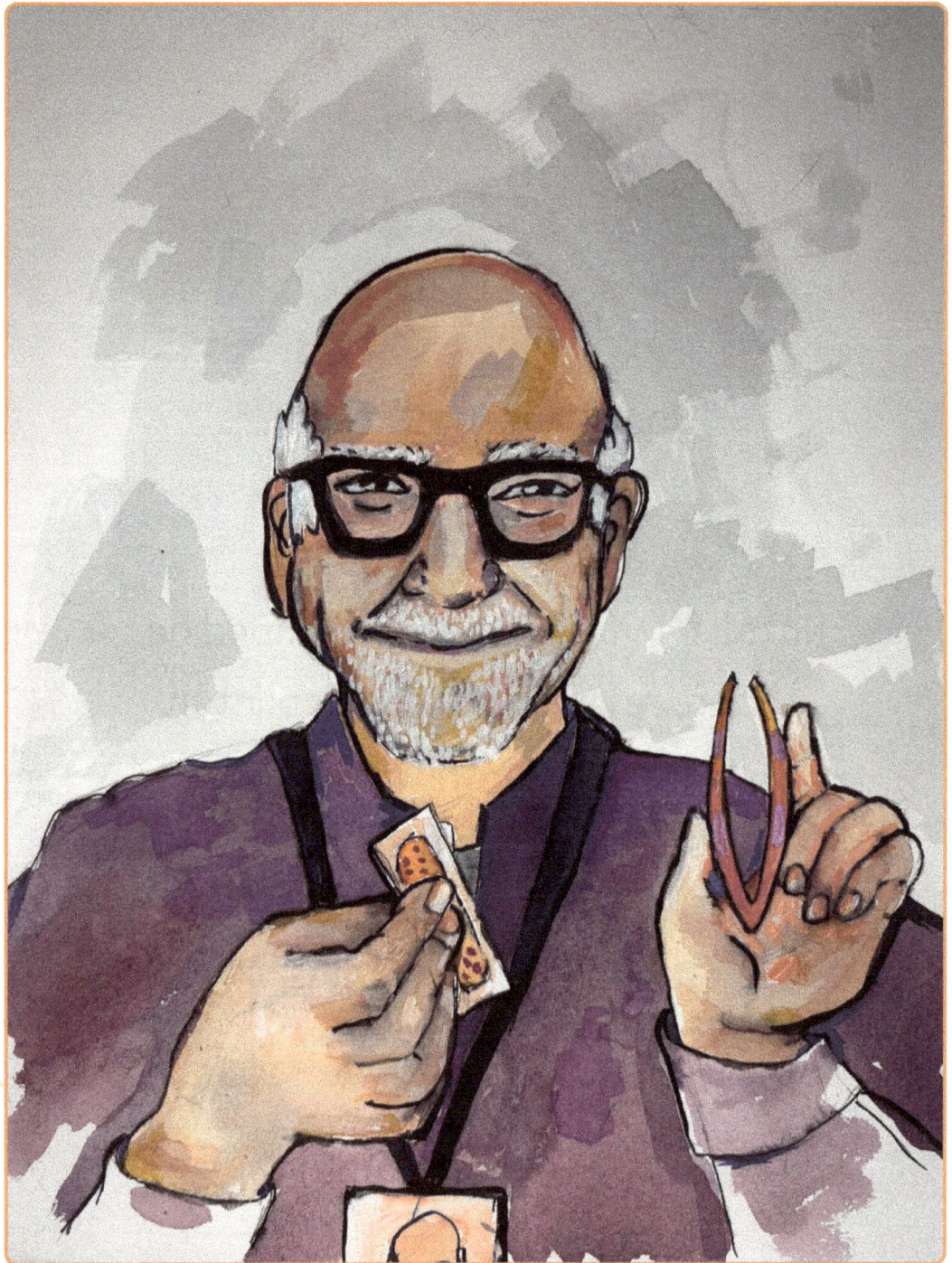

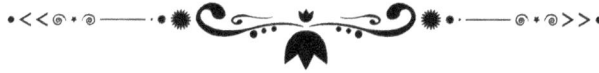

Nurse Jim nodded and asked Natalie
to sit down.

He reached into his desk drawer and
pulled out a pair of tweezers with
bright, colorful handles.

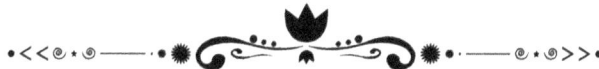

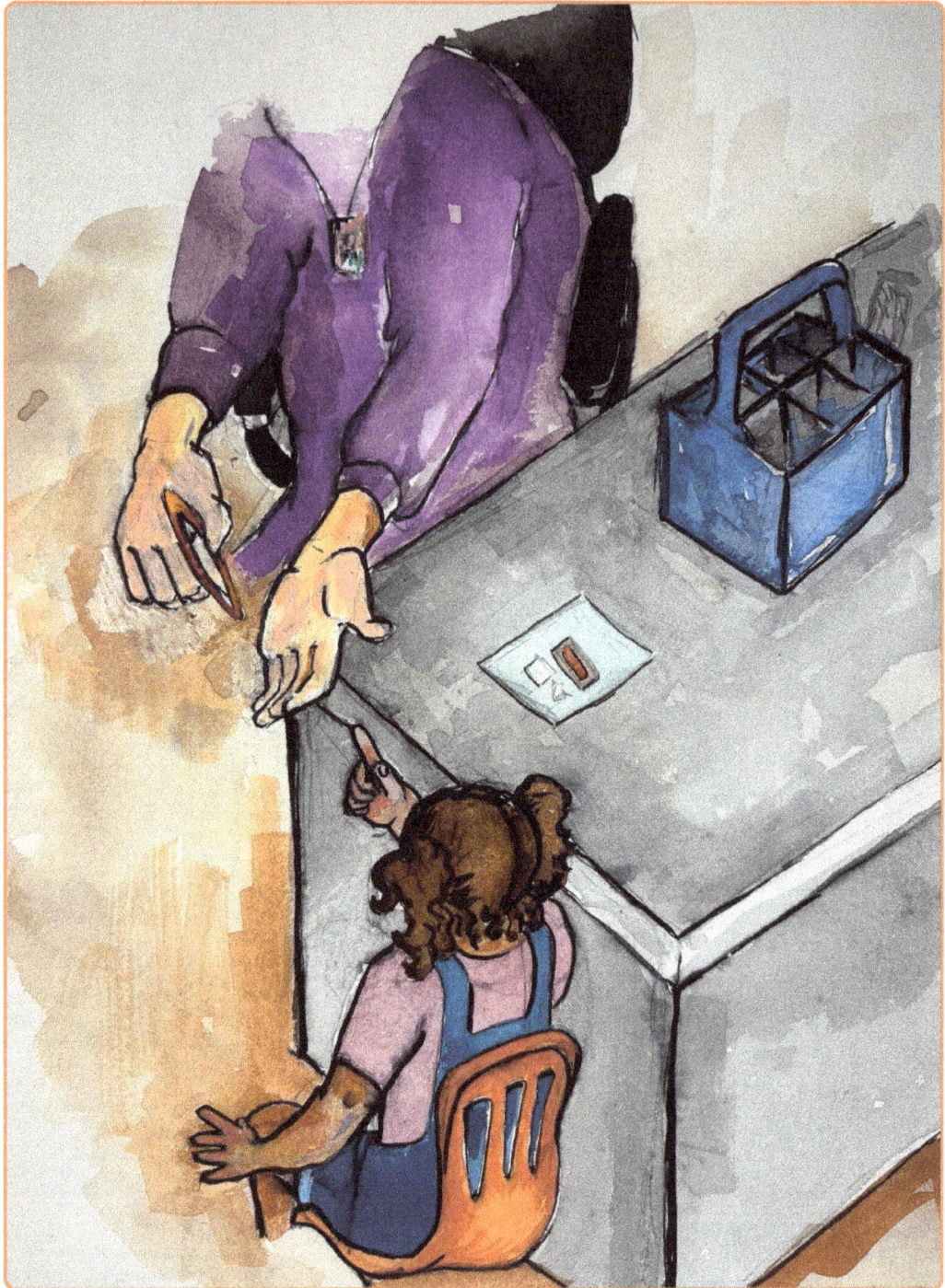

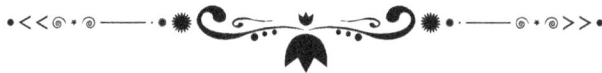

"Don't worry, Natalie. I'll have that splinter out in no time,"
Nurse Jim said with a reassuring smile.

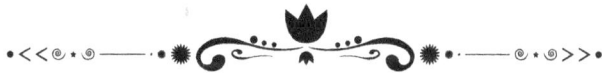

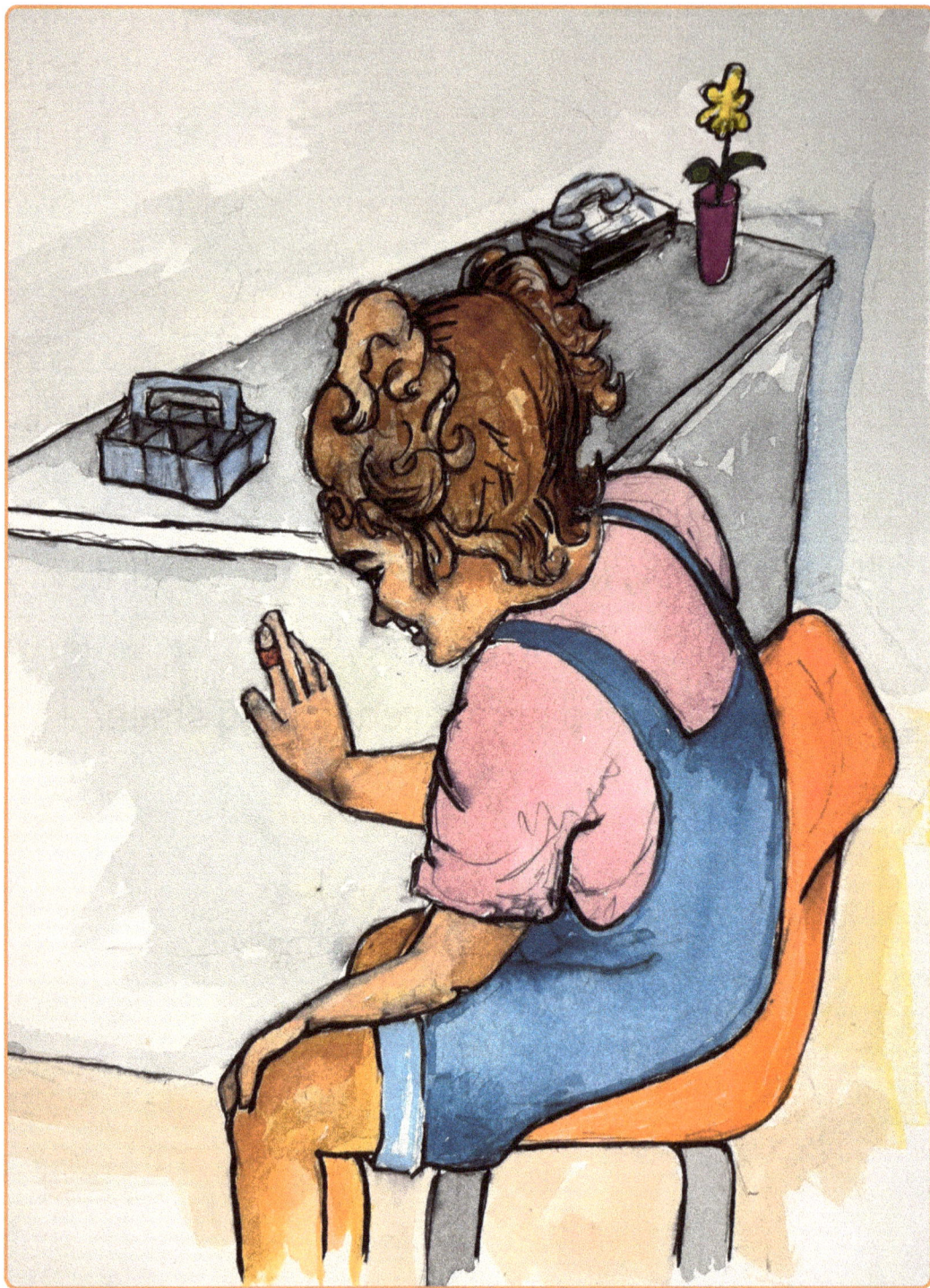

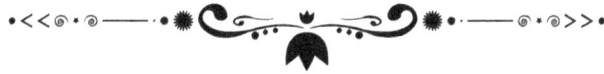

Natalie observed with astonishment
as Nurse Jim gently took out the splinter
from her finger and covered it with
a colorful band-aid.

"There, that's all better,"
Nurse Jim said with a smile.

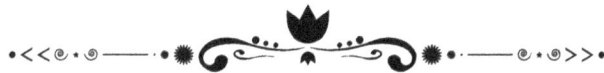

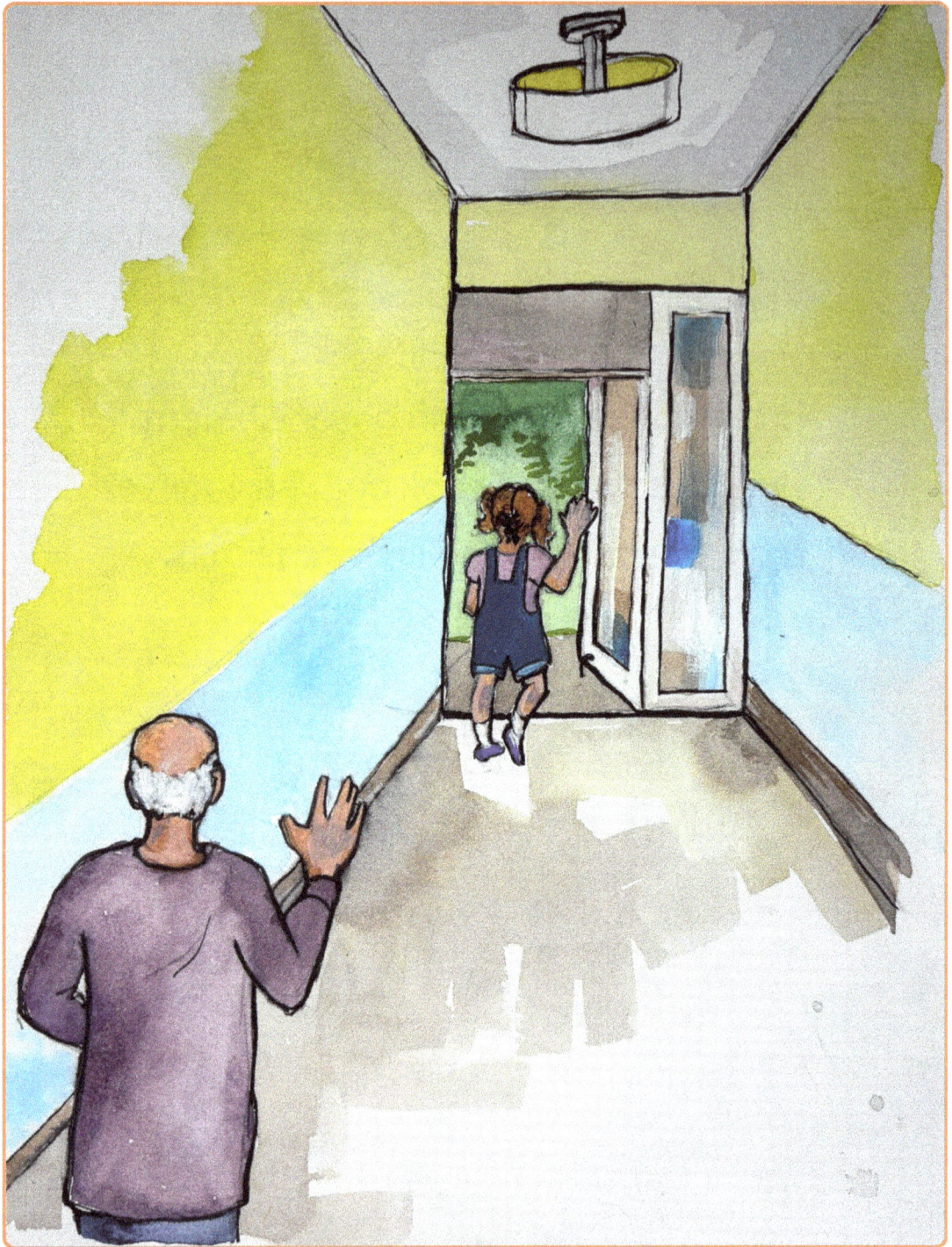

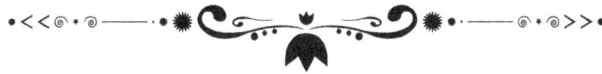

Natalie's tears changed into a smile
as she thanked Nurse Jim and
skipped back to the playground.

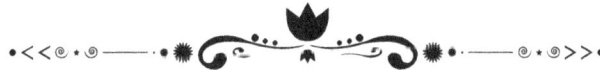

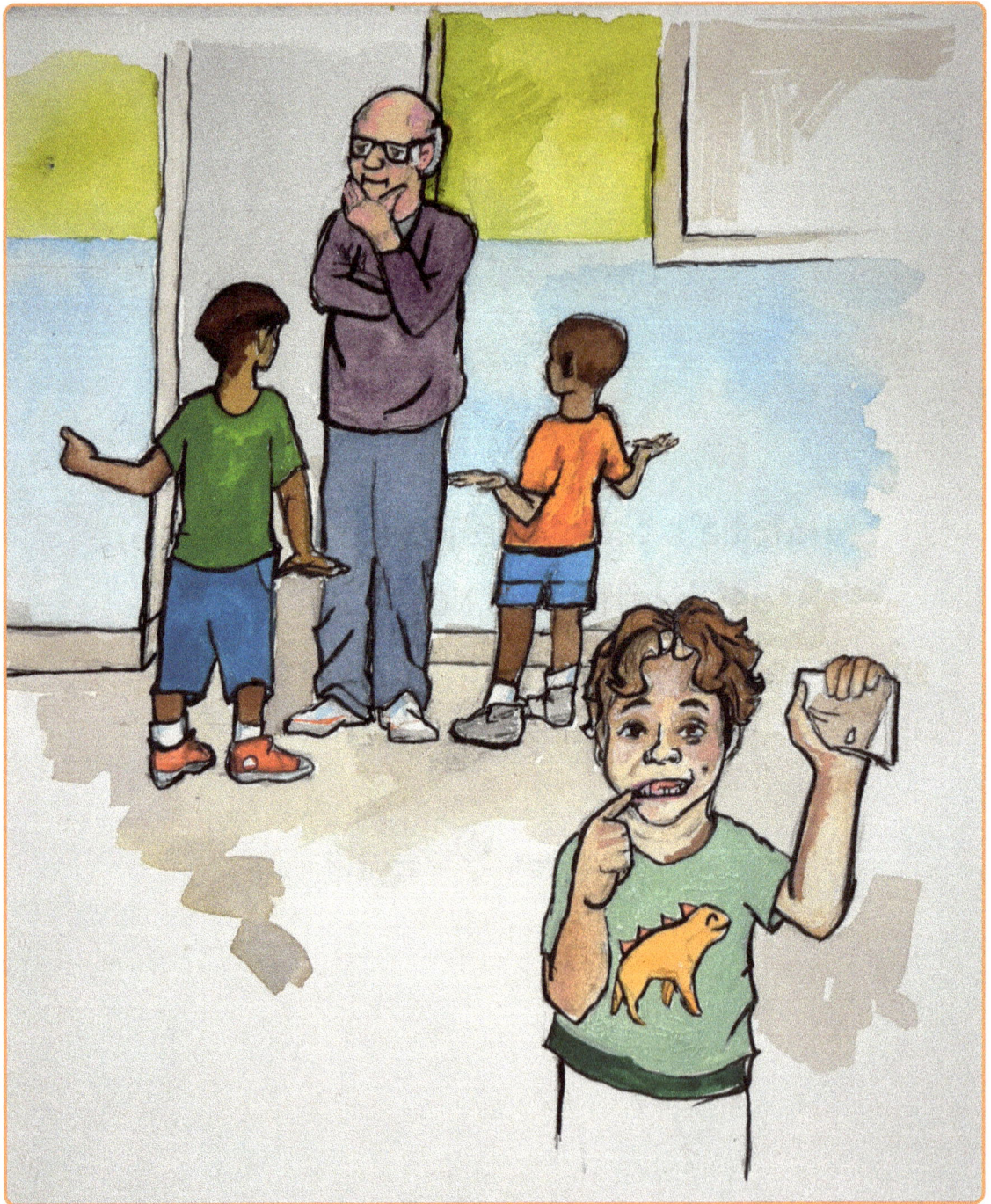

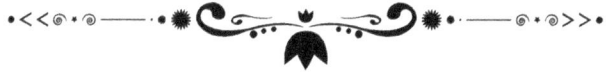

During the day, Nurse Jim cared for minor injuries and illnesses with his special touch.

He listened to tales of lost teeth, playground escapades, and fears of darkness, always providing a compassionate ear and a friendly smile.

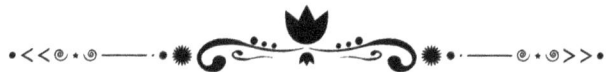

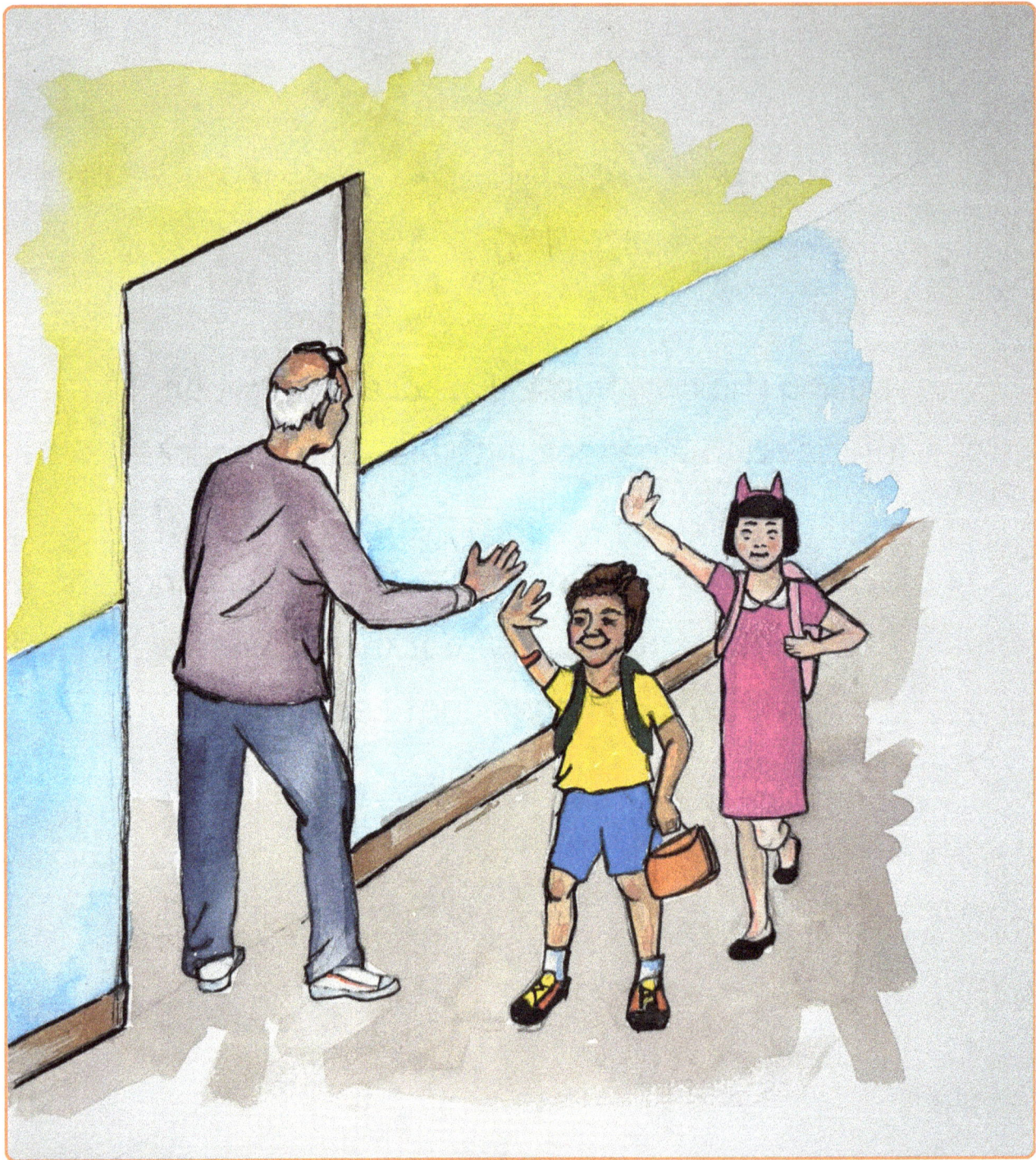

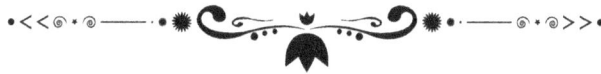

As the school day drew to a close and
the children were making their way home,
Nurse Jim stood in the hallway wishing
the students a wonderful evening.

He was aware that he had lent a helping
hand, and that was the most rewarding
part of his job.

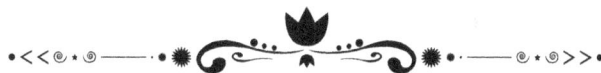

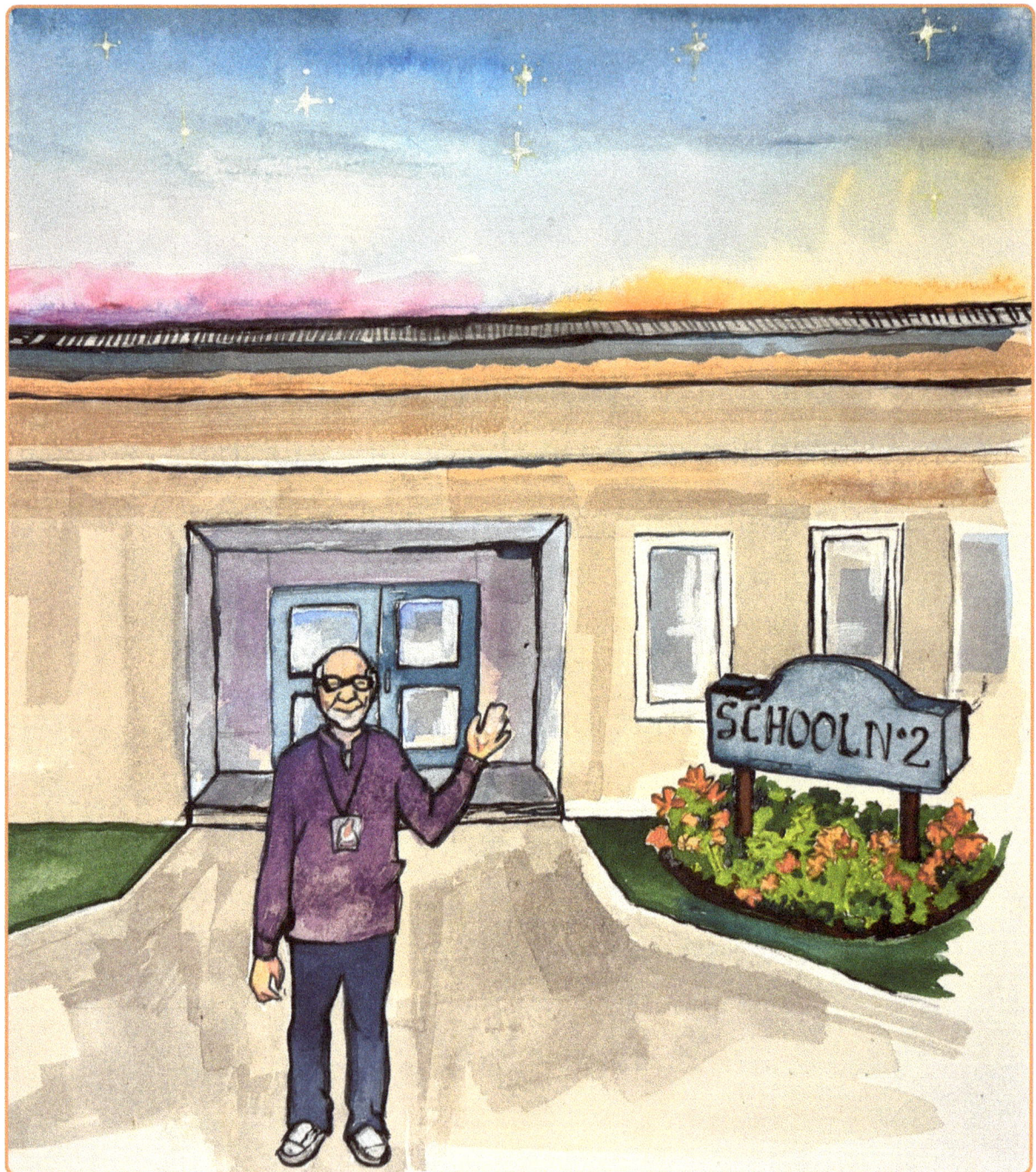

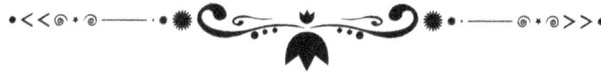

And so with the sun sinking and the stars twinkling, Nurse Jim closed his office with a smile, excited to greet the children warmly the next day and lend a helping hand to anyone in need.

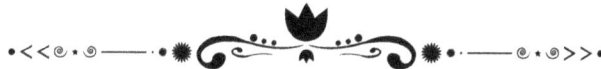

www.ingramcontent.com/pod-product-compliance
Lightning Source LLC
Chambersburg PA
CBHW080430030426
42335CB00020B/2662